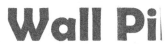 

Wall Pi|

Super Easy 10-Minute Workouts with Illustrated Exercises to Sculpt Your Body, Tone Your Muscles, and Make You Feel 15 Years Younger in Less than 28 Days

Copyright 2024- All rights reserved.
The content contained within this book may not be reproduced, duplicated or transmitted without direct written permission from the author or the publisher.
Under no circumstances will any blame or legal responsibility be held against the publisher, or author, for any damages, reparation, or monetary loss due to the information contained within this book. Either directly or indirectly.

Legal Notice:
This book is copyright protected. This book is only for personal use. You cannot amend, distribute, sell, use, quote or paraphrase any part, or the content within this book, without the consent of the author or publisher.

Disclaimer Notice: Please note the information contained within this document is for educational and entertainment purposes only. All effort has been executed to present accurate, up to date, and reliable, complete information. No warranties of any kind are declared or implied. Readers acknowledge that the author is not engaging in the rendering of legal, financial, medical or professional advice. The content within this book has been derived from various sources. Please consult a licensed professional before attempting any techniques outlined in this book.

By reading this document, the reader agrees that under no circumstances is the author responsible for any losses, direct or indirect, which are incurred as a result of the use of information contained within this document, including, but not limited to,- errors, omissions, or inaccuracies.

TABLE OF CONTENTS

INTRODUCTION..4

CHAPTER 1 - PILATES MEETS THE WALL.....................7

THE SIX PILLARS OF PILATES...7

WALL PILATES..8

BENEFITS...10

THE IMPORTANCE OF THE CORE.....................................12

CHAPTER 2 – GET READY FOR THE WORKOUT 15

PREPARE YOUR SPACE 15

WARMING UP ROUTINE 16

CHAPTER 3 – UPPER BODY EXERCISES 19

WALL PUSH-UP 19

SINGLE-ARM WALL PUSH-UP 21

WALL ANGEL..23

ROWER TO THE WALL 25

CHAPTER 4 – CORE EXERCISES..................................26

WALL PLANK..26

WALL PLANK WITH KNEE BEND 28

REVERSE WALL PLANK..30

WALL SIT 31

WALL SIT WITH KNEE RAISE..33

WALL ROLL-UPS 35

WALL TEASER..37

WALL CRUNCH 39

LATERAL WALL CRUNCH..41

WALL HUNDRED 42

CHAPTER 5 – LEG EXERCISES....................................44

Wall Squats 44

Single-Leg Squat 46

Wall Lunges 48

Wall Bridge 50

Wall Side Leg Lifts 52

Wall Calf Raises 54

Wall Scissors 56

CHAPTER 6 – POSTURE EXERCISES 58

Wall Posture Check 58

Wall Clock 60

Wall Toe Lift 62

Wall March 64

CHAPTER 7 – FLEXIBILITY EXERCISES 66

Hamstring Stretch Against the Wall 66

Chest Stretch 68

Wall Leg Swings 70

Wall Spine Stretch 72

Shoulder Stretch Against the Wall 74

Knee to Chest Stretch 75

CHAPTER 8 – 28-DAY CHALLENGE 77

How it works 77

Week 1 80

Week 2 83

Week 3 86

Week 4 89

BONUS CHAPTER- BREATHING AND RELAXATION TECHNIQUES 92

EXTRA CONTENT 101

Introduction

Welcome to a transformative journey with "Wall Pilates" – a guide designed to lead you through a precise and simple regimen that will not only reshape your body and tone your muscles but also rejuvenate your spirit. This book is more than just a compilation of exercises; it's a comprehensive approach to enhancing your overall health and well-being, both mentally and physically.

Pilates, a method known for its effectiveness in building strength, flexibility, and mindfulness, has been adapted in this book to be practiced with just one simple prop – a wall. This adaptation makes it accessible and practical for everyone, regardless of their fitness level or experience with Pilates.

This book emphasizes the importance of mental health and its interconnection with physical fitness. The exercises are curated not only to improve physical appearance, loose weight and tone the muscles, but also to instill a sense of mental clarity and peace. The practice of Wall Pilates will not only make you feel younger and more energetic but will also enhance your mental resilience, leaving you more grounded and centered in your everyday life.

Book Structure

1. **Introduction to the World of Pilates:** The book opens with an engaging introduction to the fascinating world of Pilates providing a foundational understanding that enhances the practical application of the exercises.

2. **Practical Tips for Muscle Activation:** Early in the book, we delve into practical tips and techniques to activate the muscles effectively, including pre and post-workout strategies, vital for preparing the body for exercise and aiding recovery afterward. These practices are designed to optimize your workout sessions and ensure safety and efficacy.

3. **Relaxation and Proper Breathing Techniques:** Recognizing the integral role of relaxation and breathing in Pilates, this section is dedicated to teaching proper breathing methods and relaxation techniques. This is crucial as we aim for a holistic improvement in health. Understanding and mastering these aspects are key to enhancing the effectiveness of Pilates exercises and achieving the desired results.

4. **Comprehensive Collection of Wall Pilates Exercises:** The core of the book presents an extensive collection of wall Pilates exercises. Each exercise is detailed with step-by-step instructions and accompanied by illustrative pictures. The exercises are organized into 5 main categories, allowing you to easily navigate and select exercises based on the specific muscles you want to target or the particular goals of your workout session.

5. **The 28-Day Challenge:** A pivotal feature of the book is the 28-day challenge. Although you have the flexibility to choose and mix any of the described exercises in any order you like (this is the beauty of Pilates – whichever sequence you perform, they always bring extraordinary benefits to

your body and well-being!), we have carefully curated a sequence of exercises to be performed daily, complete with detailed workout sheets. This challenge is specifically designed to maximize the benefits of wall Pilates, accelerating your journey towards achieving your health and fitness goals.

Embark on this journey with an open mind and a committed heart, and let this book be your guide to a healthier, happier you!

Do you want to access fantastic extra content ready for you to download?

Scan the QR-code or follow the link below to access everything:

https://www.readingroadspress.com/wall-pilates-bonus

- Guided meditations
- Relaxing Music
- Nature sounds for anxiety relief
- ...and much more!

Chapter 1 - Pilates Meets the Wall

Before we delve into the magic of Wall Pilates, let's rewind and explore the roots of this timeless discipline. Pilates, formulated by Joseph Pilates in the twentieth century, arises from the belief that mental and physical health are interconnected, and that control of the body can be achieved through his technique known as "Contrology." At the heart of Pilates, we find an invitation to rediscover the harmony of movement, the balance of the mind, and the synergy of muscles, through exercises that emphasize quality over quantity, precision, and fluidity.

The Six Pillars of Pilates

Traditional Pilates is built upon 6 key principles, which should be considered as intertwined threads of the same rope, all essential for the integrity and effectiveness of the practice:

1. **Concentration:** Every movement in Pilates demands complete focus, guiding awareness towards the body and the present moment.
2. **Control:** Each gesture is controlled, aiming to execute the movement with maximum efficiency and minimal effort.
3. **Centering:** The 'powerhouse' or core is the source from which strength and stability flow; it's the core of the body, including the abdomen, hips, buttocks, and back.

4. **Flow:** Movements in Pilates flow in a seamless and harmonious sequence, ensuring elegance and continuity between positions.
5. **Precision:** Each position is designed to achieve maximum benefit, with an emphasis on the correctness of form.
6. **Breath:** Breathing in Pilates is intentional and synchronized with movements, contributing to the effectiveness of exercises and concentration.

Wall Pilates

Wall Pilates is a refined extension of this practice, incorporating a fixed and stable element: the wall. This innovative fusion not only amplifies the principles of traditional Pilates but also opens up a new horizon of possibilities and benefits.

Stability and Support
- Physical Guidance: The wall serves as a physical reference point, helping maintain proper alignment during exercise.
- Enhanced Balance: The wall offers stable support that can be especially useful for beginners who are still learning to control and balance their bodies.

Resistance and Intensification
- Added Resistance: Some movements can be performed against the immovable resistance of the wall, which can help build strength and endurance.

- Intensity Variation: The distance from the wall can be used to increase or decrease the intensity of an exercise, making the workout more versatile.

Safety and Adaptability
- Reduced Risk of Injuries: For those with balance issues or specific physical conditions, the wall provides support that can reduce the risk of falls and injuries.
- Adaptability: Wall Pilates can be tailored for people of all ages and fitness levels, providing a safe option for seniors or those recovering from injuries.

Kinesthetic Feedback
- Immediate Sensation: Contact with the wall provides immediate feedback on body positioning and orientation in space, which is essential for learning proprioception and motor control.
- Posture Correction: The wall helps detect and correct asymmetries in the body, leading to greater symmetry and alignment over time.

Innovation and Variation
- Exploring New Poses: With the help of the wall, you can explore new variations of exercises that wouldn't be possible without this point of support.
- Maintaining Interest: Introducing the wall into your Pilates routine can offer a new dimension of mental and physical stimulation, keeping the workout fresh and interesting.

Focus and Concentration

- Reduced Distraction: The physical presence of the wall can help limit visual distractions, allowing the individual to better focus on their body and movement.

Benefits

Pilates offers a full range of benefits, touching on both physical and mental health. Integrating the wall into your Pilates practice can help maximize these benefits, making the practice more accessible, varied, and challenging. It's like adding a new spice to your favorite recipe!

Physical Benefits

- **Improved Core Strength:** The core is often referred to as the Pilates powerhouse. Strengthening it builds a more robust foundation for your body, enhancing stability and support throughout, thereby reducing the risk of injuries. Think of the wall as your steadfast gym companion, offering constant resistance to intensify core activation. It's like having an invisible coach encouraging you to do just one more sit-up!
- **Increased Flexibility:** Pilates promotes muscle tension release and increases muscle length, helping to prevent injuries and aches. Think of it as giving your muscles a much-needed stretch. The wall's support lets you explore new angles and movement ranges, leading to a flexibility boost.
- **Improved Posture:** With a focus on spinal position and strengthening postural muscles, Pilates helps develop better and healthier posture. Stand tall, stand proud!

- **Muscle Toning:** Unlike strength training that often builds bulkier muscles, Pilates tones muscles, making them longer and leaner. It's like sculpting your body into a work of art.
- **Improved Breathing:** Pilates encourages a pattern of deep, controlled breathing, improving circulation and promoting greater relaxation. Breathe in, breathe out, and feel the calm.
- **Balance and Coordination:** Through exercises that challenge balancing and precision, Pilates significantly improves coordination and balance. It's like training to be a tightrope walker, but safer.

Mental Benefits

- **Concentration:** Pilates requires deep mental focus to execute movements precisely, thereby improving overall attention. It's a brain workout!
- **Stress Reduction:** Thanks to the emphasis on breathing and concentration, Pilates can have a calming effect on the mind, reducing stress and anxiety. It's like meditation in motion.
- **Body Awareness:** Pilates increases awareness of one's body and how it moves in space (proprioception), improving confidence in daily and sporting movements. Become the master of your body!

Preventive and Therapeutic Benefits

- **Injury Prevention:** By strengthening the core and improving flexibility and posture, Pilates can help prevent future injuries. It's like giving your body an armor shield.
- **Injury Recovery:** Often used in rehabilitation, Pilates can be customized to fit an individual's recovery needs, helping to rebuild strength without excessive stress on the body. It's like physical therapy with a twist.

Aesthetic Benefits
- **More Sculpted and Defined Body:** With regular practice, Pilates can help build a more toned and slender figure. Get ready to rock those jeans!
- **Improved Body Composition:** Pilates can help reduce body fat and increase lean muscle mass. It's like a natural body sculpting tool.

The Importance of the Core

The term "core" refers to the group of muscles forming the body's central area, including the abdominal muscles, lower back muscles, pelvic muscles, and some hip muscles. It's important to train the core because it acts as a central point of strength for the entire body and plays a crucial role in numerous functions:

1. **Spinal Support:** The core stabilizes the spine, reducing the risk of back injuries and pain. It's like having an internal back brace.
2. **Posture Improvement:** Strong core muscles keep the body upright and aligned, contributing to better posture. Stand like a proud peacock!

3. **Movement Efficiency:** A trained core allows for more efficient and powerful movements, both in daily life and sports. It's like upgrading your body's engine.
4. **Balance and Stability:** A strong core helps maintain balance, especially during movements that involve changes in direction or position. It's the secret to not toppling over.
5. **Injury Prevention:** Strengthening the core is essential in preventing injuries, particularly those related to sports and physical activity. It's your body's natural insurance policy.
6. **Athletic Performance Improvement:** The core is involved in virtually all types of sports movements; thus, a strong core can improve overall athletic performance. Play like a pro!
7. **Daily Functionality:** Daily actions, like lifting objects or even standing, require the use of the core. It's the hero behind your everyday activities.

Pilates is crucial for core training. Most exercises emphasize movements originating from the body's center, training the core consistently and intentionally. It's like targeting your body's command center.

- **Balance Between Strength and Flexibility:** Pilates focuses not just on muscle strength but also on flexibility, ensuring a balanced workout that avoids muscle overloads.
- **Control and Precision:** Many Pilates exercises require a high degree of control and precision, which are essential for correctly activating core muscles.

- **Breathing:** Pilates teaches breathing techniques that encourage core activation and its proper use during exercises. Breathe your way to a stronger core!
- **Low-Impact Exercises:** The low-impact nature of Pilates makes it suitable for individuals of all fitness levels, allowing anyone to build core strength without risking joint health.
- **Mind-Body Connection:** Pilates requires a mind-body connection that helps develop awareness of how the core muscles are activated and used during exercise.

In summary, the core is the body's center of strength that supports and facilitates all its movements. Pilates is particularly effective in strengthening the core because it incorporates targeted exercises that emphasize control, precision, and correct breathing, all key elements for an effective core workout.

Chapter 2 – Get Ready for the Workout

Prepare Your Space

The first step on this wall Pilates adventure is creating a space that not only welcomes your practice but nurtures it. Let's discover how to set up the ideal spot for our wall Pilates routine.

Choosing the Right Place

The location choice is crucial. You need a calm environment where concentration and tranquility can blossom. It could be a corner of your living room, a dedicated room, or any space that can be converted for this purpose. The key is having enough room to move freely and unrestrictedly. Imagine a space where your limbs can stretch and twirl without knocking over your favorite vase!

Creating a Serene Environment

The atmosphere should be relaxing. Consider using soft colors for the walls that don't distract but invite concentration. The lighting should be gentle, yet bright enough to clearly see your movements without straining your eyes. Think of a cozy nook that whispers, "Let's do Pilates!"

Wall Space

The wall will be your partner during the Pilates practice. Choose a wall free from paintings, furniture, or other objects that could interfere with your movements or cause harm if bumped into. The wall's surface should be smooth to ensure safe and stable contact during exercises. It's like finding the perfect dance partner who won't step on your toes!

The Mat

The mat is another crucial element. It should be thick enough to protect your joints but also grippy enough to prevent slipping. Choose a high-quality one because it will be the foundation for your exercises and support you throughout the practice.

Warming Up Routine

A thorough warm-up not only increases the efficiency of your wall Pilates practice but also helps to prevent injuries, making the body more receptive to the subsequent exercises. Remember to listen to your body and gradually increase the intensity of the warm-up exercises. With your body and mind adequately prepared, you're now ready to face an effective and satisfying wall Pilates session.

1. Breathing and Centering

Start with a few minutes of deep breathing, sitting or standing near the wall. Close your eyes and focus on your breath. Inhale deeply through your nose, expanding your diaphragm, and exhale slowly through your mouth, feeling your body relax. This breathing helps center your mind and connect with your "powerhouse," the energetic center of Pilates.

2. Neck and Shoulder Mobilization

After breathing, move on to mobilizing your neck and shoulders. Gently rotate your head from one shoulder to the other, then perform small circles with your shoulders, first forwards and then backwards. Place your hands on the wall and, keeping your feet slightly apart, lean slightly forward and push your chest towards the wall to open your shoulders and chest.

3. Warming Up Arms and Legs

Continue with dynamic exercises for arms and legs. Stand an arm's length from the wall, place your hands on the wall, and alternate dynamic pushes, as if you were doing vertical push-ups. Then, turn your back to the wall and, with your hands resting on it, perform light knee bends to warm up your legs.

4. Spine Mobilization

The health of the spine is essential in Pilates. Stand with your back to the wall, feet slightly apart, and slowly slide down the wall, vertebra by vertebra, until you reach an imaginary seated position. Stand up again with the same control. This exercise helps to become aware of individual vertebrae and improve back mobility.

5. Warming Up Hips and Ankles

Move on to your hips and ankles. Lean one hip against the wall and laterally lift the free leg, maintaining control and without swaying. Then, with wall support, perform ankle circles to increase joint mobility.

6. Core Activation

The core is the focal point of Pilates. With your shoulders against the wall, alternately lift your knees as if you were marching on the spot, focusing on activating the core with each lift. Then perform some "roll downs," i.e., rolling down the spine towards the floor, starting from the head and unrolling until you touch the floor with your fingertips, then rise again with the same control.

7. Exercises for Joint Mobility

Incorporate specific exercises for the mobility of the main joints, such as the pelvis and shoulders. Perform pelvis rotations, maintaining contact with the wall, and arm circumductions, resting your hand on the wall and moving your arm in large circles to warm up the shoulder joint.

8. Dynamic Stretching

Finish the warm-up with dynamic stretches. Lean sideways against the wall and reach up with the other arm, leaning your torso and feeling a stretch on the side of your body. Alternatively, you can perform gentle twists of the torso with your hands on the wall, to prepare the spine for more complex movements.

Chapter 3 – Upper Body Exercises

Wall Push-Up

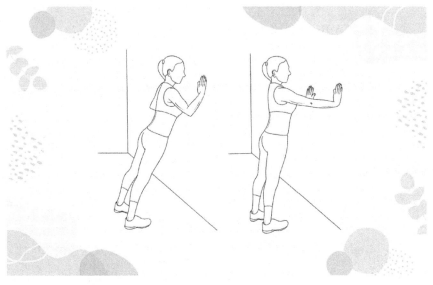

Positioning

1. **Initial Position:** Stand at an arm's length away from the wall. Extend your arms in front of you and press your flat palms against the wall, about shoulder-width apart. Imagine giving the wall a high-five for being a loyal supporter of your fitness journey.

2. **Foot Position:** Keep your feet hip-width apart.

3. **Posture Check:** Maintain your body in a straight line from your head to heels. Picture balancing a book on your head. Let's not let it fall, shall we?

The Exercise

1. **Bend and Extend:** Inhale as you bend your elbows to bring your chest closer to the wall. Visualize yourself as a human accordion, or if you prefer, as if you were about to give a kiss to that beautiful wall in front of you.

2. **The Push:** Exhale as you push back to the starting position. Use the strength of your arms and chest as if you were pushing open a heavy door. But remember, no cheating: keep your body as straight as a plank.

Variations

- **Narrow Hand Position:** For working on your triceps, simply bring your hands closer on the wall.

- **Single Leg Lift:** For an extra challenge, lift one leg off the ground while performing the push-up. Keep alternating. Who says we can't multitask?

Safety Notes

1. **Keep Your Core Engaged:** Keep your core active throughout the exercise to protect your back. If your back starts to curve like a grumpy cat, you're losing form.

2. **Elbow Alignment:** Make sure your elbows don't flare out too much; keep them a bit close to your body. You're doing push-ups, not trying to fly!

Single-Arm Wall Push-Up

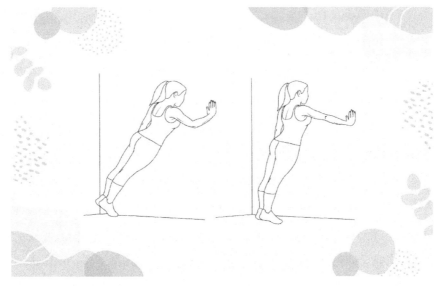

This exercise is a bit more challenging than the standard wall push-up, so prepare yourself mentally.

Initial Positioning

1. **Distance from the Wall:** Stand about an arm's length away from the wall.
2. **One Hand on the Wall:** Place one hand flat against the wall, while the other hand is on your hip or behind your back.
3. **Feet Alignment:** Ensure your feet are parallel and aligned with your hips.
4. **Posture:** Keep your spine straight and your core active.

Performing the Exercise

1. **Downward Phase:** Inhale deeply and start to bend your elbow while keeping your hand firmly against the wall. As in

21

the standard wall push-up, aim to bring your chest closer to the wall. It's like a hug, but with the wall. Romantic, right?

2. **Push Phase:** Exhale and push with your arm to return to the starting position. Imagine pushing away all your worries with that single powerful hand.

Remember

-   **Keep Your Core Engaged:** Always, always, always. This helps maintain proper posture and protect your back.
-   **Elbow Close to Your Body:** Even when using one arm, keep the elbow close to your body to avoid unnecessary strain.

Wall Angel

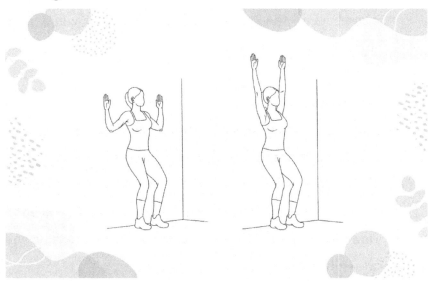

Initial Positioning

1. **Close to the Wall:** Stand close to the wall so that your back, buttocks, and heels touch it.

2. **Arms on the Wall:** Lift your arms and place them against the wall, forming a 90-degree angle at your elbows.

3. **Alignment:** Ensure your head, back, and buttocks maintain contact with the wall throughout the exercise.

Performing the Exercise

1. **Ascending Phase:** Inhale slowly and begin to raise your arms along the wall, always keeping contact. Imagine you are an angel spreading its wings. Isn't that poetic?

2. **Maximum Extension:** Try to extend your arms as much as possible without lifting your elbows or hands off the wall. At this moment, you are an angel in all its glory!

3. **Descending Phase:** Exhale and slowly begin to lower your arms back to the starting position, as if your wings were tired after a long flight.

Points to Remember

- **Constant Contact:** Always maintain contact with the wall. This is the secret to correctly performing the exercise.
- **Active Core:** Again, keep your core engaged to maintain correct posture and provide that extra stability you need.
- **Don't Overexert:** The goal is to work on mobility and strength, not to push yourself too hard.

Rower to the Wall

The "Rower to the Wall" is a unique and effective Wall Pilates exercise designed to strengthen the upper body, particularly targeting the back, shoulders, and arms, while also engaging the core muscles. The exercise mimics the motion of rowing, but is performed against a wall, providing resistance and stability.

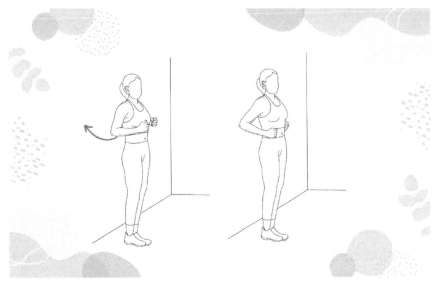

Put your back against the wall. with your feet hip-width apart. In the initial phase the back is supported against the wall.

At the beginning the arms can be stretched along the body or bent with the elbows resting on the wall. During the traction phase you must push your elbows against the wall, pulling your chest out and, consequently, detaching your back from the wall.

Slowly return to the starting position and repeat the exercise.

Inhale as you push away from the wall.

Exhale as you return to the starting position.

Chapter 4 — Core Exercises

Wall Plank

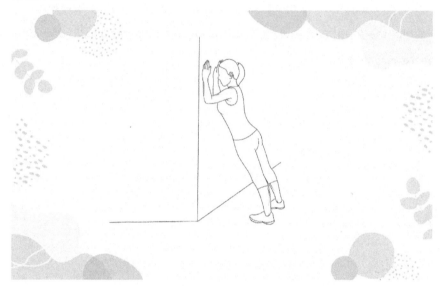

A Fantastic Way to Strengthen Your Core and Upper Body. Start with 30 seconds and gradually increase the duration as you get stronger. This exercise is ideal for everyone, from Pilates beginners to seasoned veterans!

Initial Positioning

1. **Distance from the Wall:** Approach the wall and place your hands on it at shoulder height.
2. **Feet Backward:** Take a couple of steps back until your body forms a straight line from your feet to your head.
3. **Open Hands:** Your hands should be aligned with your shoulders, and your palms should firmly adhere to the wall.

Performing the Exercise

1. **Preparation:** Engage your core and ensure your body is in a straight line. Activate your abs and relax your shoulders.
2. **Holding the Position:** Maintain this position, making sure your belly doesn't sag and your buttocks don't lift up.
3. **Breathing:** Breathe deeply, aiming to hold the position for at least 30 seconds or as long as you can.
4. **Relaxation:** After completing, walk your feet towards the wall and release the position.

Points to Remember

- **Keep the Core Active:** This is crucial for correct exercise execution and to prevent overloading the lower back.
- **Don't Lock Your Knees:** Keep them slightly bent to avoid strain.

Safety Tips

- Avoid this exercise if you have back or shoulder issues unless approved by a health professional.

Wall Plank with Knee Bend

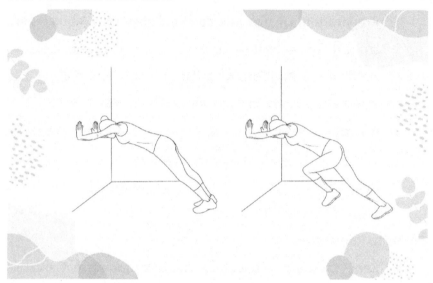

This is an advanced Wall Plank variation that not only strengthens your core but also your leg muscles. Start with a few repetitions and increase as you become more comfortable with the exercise.

Initial Positioning

1. **Distance from the Wall:** Approach the wall and place your hands on it at shoulder height.
2. **Feet Backward:** Take a couple of steps back until your body is inclined and forms a straight line from your feet to your head.
3. **Open Hands:** Your hands should be aligned with your shoulders, and your palms must adhere well to the wall.

Performing the Exercise

1. **Preparation:** Engage your core and stabilize your body in an inclined plank position.

2. **Knee Tuck:** Lift one knee towards your chest while maintaining the plank position. Return to the starting position.

3. **Switch Sides:** Repeat the movement with the other knee.

4. **Breathing:** Keep your breathing smooth and deep throughout the exercise.

5. **Repetitions:** Aim for at least 10-15 repetitions per side, or as comfortable.

6. **Relaxation:** After completing, walk your feet towards the wall and release the position.

Points to Remember

- **Maintain Core Engagement:** This is essential to protect the lower back and enhance exercise effectiveness.
- **Don't Lock Your Knees:** Keep them slightly bent to avoid overloading the joints.

Reverse Wall Plank

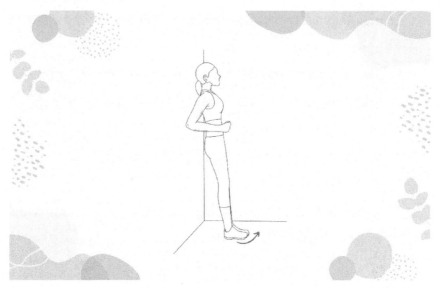

In the reverse plank, you will position yourself opposite to the classic plank. That means your back will be towards the wall. Take a few steps forward, then lean on the wall with your elbows (similar to the wall row exercise position). Your heels are on the ground, but your feet are slightly angled upwards. Hold the position for a few seconds.

Wall Sit

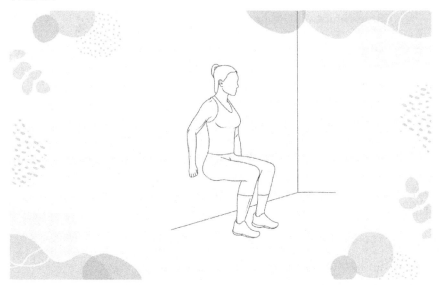

The "Wall Sit" is an excellent exercise for strengthening not just the core, but also the quadriceps and glutes.

1. **Initial Position:** Place your back against a wall with your feet shoulder-width apart and step forward a few paces from the wall.

2. **Lowering Down:** Slowly lower yourself until your thighs are parallel to the ground, as if sitting on an invisible chair. Your body should form a 90-degree angle at the knees.

3. **Alignment:** Ensure your knees are directly above your ankles and not extending beyond your toes. Your shoulders and back should remain flat against the wall.

4. **Arm Position:** Keep your arms extended along your body or crossed on your chest to avoid leaning on your thighs.

5. **Holding the Position:** Hold this position, keeping your abdominal muscles contracted to support your back.

6. **Breathing:** Focus on regular and controlled breathing to help maintain the position.

7. **Duration:** The goal is to stay in this seated position for at least 30 seconds, but with practice, aim to gradually increase up to 1-2 minutes.

8. **Rest and Repeat:** Slowly rise up and rest for 30 seconds. Repeat the exercise 3-5 times.

Tips:

- **For Beginners:** Start with short intervals of 10-15 seconds and gradually increase the duration.
- **For Intermediate:** Maintain the position for 45-60 seconds.
- **For Advanced:** Try holding the position for over 1 minute or add weight to increase intensity.

Wall Sit with Knee Raise

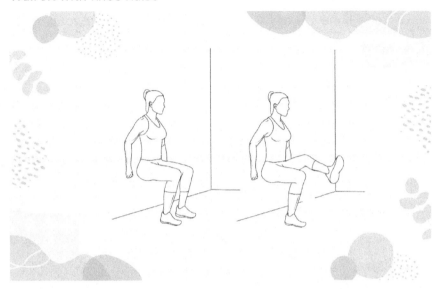

The "Wall Sit with Knee Raise" combines the benefits of a classic wall sit with more intense work on the abdominal muscles and hip mobility. It's a great way to increase the difficulty of the standard exercise and further engage the core.

1. **Initial Position:** Position your back against the wall with your feet shoulder-width apart and step about one and a half steps away from the wall.
2. **Lowering Down:** Slowly lower yourself until your thighs are parallel to the floor, maintaining a 90-degree angle at the knees.
3. **Alignment:** Ensure your knees are above your ankles and not beyond your toes. Keep your back flat against the wall.
4. **Arm Position:** Keep your arms extended along your body or crossed on your chest.

5. **Holding and Knee Raise:** While in the wall sit position, lift one knee toward your chest without moving your upper body, then lower it back down with control. Repeat with the other leg.

6. **Breathing:** Maintain controlled and deep breathing throughout the exercise.

7. **Duration and Repetitions:** Alternate legs for 10 lifts per leg, maintaining the base position of the wall sit throughout.

8. **Rest and Sets:** After completing the repetitions on both legs, slowly rise to rest. Rest for 30-60 seconds and repeat for 2-3 sets.

Tips:

- Start with a reduced number of repetitions and sets, gradually increasing as your strength and endurance improve.
- **For Beginners:** Perform the movement slowly and with a reduced number of repetitions.
- **For Intermediate:** Add more repetitions and hold the position longer.
- **For Advanced:** Consider using ankle weights to increase resistance.

Wall Roll-Ups

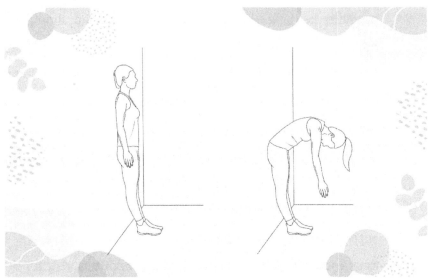

"Wall Roll-Ups" help improve spinal mobility, hamstring flexibility, and core strength. This exercise also aids in promoting body awareness and movement control, central elements in Pilates.

1. **Initial Position:** Stand with your back to the wall, feet shoulder-width apart and slightly away from the wall, arms extended in front of you.

2. **Start of Roll Down:** Slowly begin to "unroll" your spine from the head down, vertebra by vertebra, tucking your head and sliding your hands down the wall.

3. **Sliding Down:** As you lower yourself, let your hands slide down the wall, allowing your torso to bend forward and your hips to flex.

4. **Bent Position:** Continue until your hands touch the floor, if possible, keeping your legs straight. Your head should be between your arms, facing your knees.

5. **Roll Up:** Slowly begin to rise back up, "rolling" your spine up against the wall, vertebra by vertebra, until you return to an upright position.

6. **Breathing:** Inhale as you lower down and exhale as you rise, matching the movement to your breath's rhythm.

7. **Duration and Repetitions:** Perform the exercise slowly and with control for 5-10 repetitions.

8. **Rest and Sets:** After completing the repetitions, rest for 30 seconds and repeat for 2-3 sets.

Wall Teaser

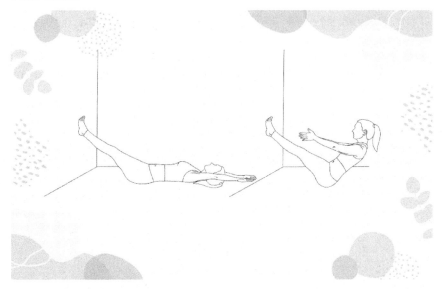

An Advanced Exercise for Core Strength, Coordination, and Balance
This wall version provides guidance for proper leg alignment and supports the core during the lifting and lowering of the body.

1. **Initial Position:** Lie down with your back on the floor, lift your legs and place your feet flat against the wall. Your back should be straight, and your arms extended in front of you, parallel to the floor.
2. **Lift:** Exhale, keeping your legs against the wall, lift your arms and torso towards the ceiling, tilting your pelvis until your body forms a 'V' shape.
3. **Teaser Position:** Once in position, your legs are straight with heels against the wall, arms extended towards your feet.

4. **Control and Balance:** Hold the position for a moment, finding balance and controlling the movement with your core.

5. **Return:** Inhale and slowly start bringing your torso and arms back to the floor, simultaneously bending your knees and bringing your feet back against the wall.

6. **Repetitions:** Perform the exercise for 3-5 repetitions.

7. **Duration:** Hold the 'V' position for 3-5 deep breaths each time.

Tips:

- Keep the core active throughout to support the back and control the movement.
- Move slowly and with control, especially when returning to the initial position.
- If the movement is too challenging, start by bending your knees more.

Wall Crunch

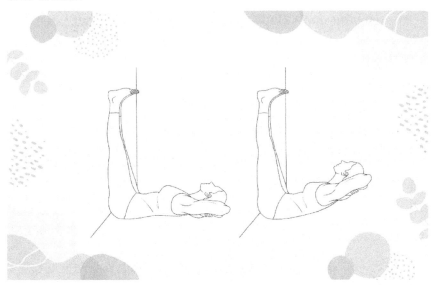

A Great Exercise for Targeting the Abs Safely and Effectively Using the wall not only helps maintain the correct leg position but also provides slight resistance that can increase the exercise's intensity for the abs without overloading the back.

1. **Initial Position:** Lie on the floor close to the wall, with legs lifted and entirely resting against it. (Alternatively, you can keep your legs bent at a 90-degree angle with your feet against the wall.) Your back should be in contact with the floor, and your hands positioned behind your head or crossed on your chest.

2. **Core Activation:** Engage your core by contracting your abdominal muscles. This helps protect your back and adds strength to the movement.

3. **Lifting:** Inhale to prepare for the movement. As you exhale, lift your upper body towards your knees, keeping your neck relaxed and your chin slightly away from your chest.

4. **Return:** Inhale and slowly lower your back to the floor, controlling the movement with your abs.

5. **Repetitions:** Perform 10 to 15 repetitions per set.

6. **Sets:** Complete 2 to 3 sets, with a rest of 30-60 seconds between each set.

Tips:

- Don't use your neck or arms to pull yourself up; the movement should come from the core.
- Keep the movement smooth and controlled, avoiding momentum.
- If you feel neck tension, reposition your hands to better support your head.

Lateral Wall Crunch

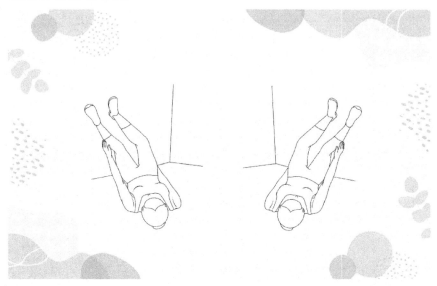

Wall Hundred

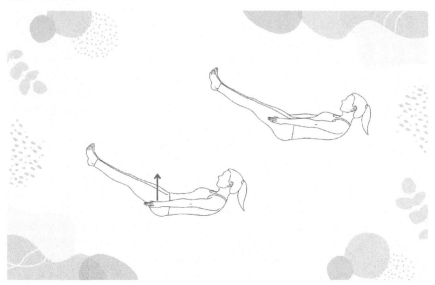

A Variation of the Classic Pilates Exercise 'The Hundred'. This exercise is designed to strengthen the core, improve circulation, and increase muscular endurance through the constant aerobic activity of arm movements combined with controlled breathing.

1. **Initial Position:** Lie on your back with legs raised and feet flat against the wall. Legs can be straight or bent at a 90-degree angle.
2. **Arm Support:** Extend your arms along the sides of your body, slightly lifting them off the ground.
3. **Core Movement:** Start activating your core, keeping your back firmly flattened on the mat without arching the lower back.

4. **Arm Pulsations:** Begin moving your arms up and down in small rhythmic pulsations, as if you were gently patting water in a pool.

5. **Breathing:** Synchronize your breath with the pulsations: inhale deeply for 5 pulsations and then exhale for another 5, maintaining core contraction.

6. **Duration:** Continue performing arm pulsations and synchronized breathing for a total of 100 counts – hence the name "Hundred."

Tips:

- Keep your chin slightly tucked towards your chest to avoid neck strain.
- The abdominal muscles should remain contracted throughout the exercise to support the spine.
- Look towards your navel to keep your neck aligned with your spine.

Duration of Each Exercise: Approximately 1-2 minutes, completing 100 counts (pulsations). It can be repeated 2-3 times within a larger workout session, with a 1-minute break between repetitions if necessary.

Chapter 5 – Leg Exercises

Wall Squats

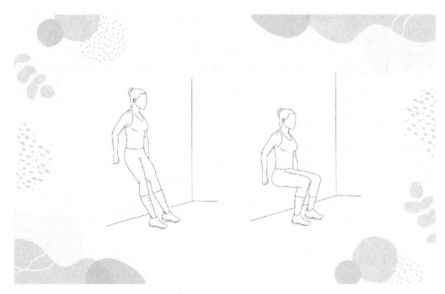

Wall Squats are an excellent exercise for toning leg muscles, glutes, and core, while also improving strength and muscular endurance. Using the wall helps maintain proper posture during the exercise and can be especially helpful for those with balance issues or who want to focus on form.

1. **Initial Position:** Stand with your back against the wall. Your feet should be shoulder-width apart and slightly forward from the wall.
2. **Descending:** Slide slowly down the wall by bending your knees, as if sitting on an invisible chair. Ensure your knees

are aligned with your ankles and don't push beyond your toes.

3. **Knee Angle:** Stop descending when your thighs are parallel to the floor, and your knees form a 90-degree angle.

4. **Holding the Position:** Maintain this position as if you are doing a "wall squat." Ensure that your core is engaged and your back is flat against the wall.

5. **Rising Up:** Push through your heels to slowly return to the initial standing position.

Tips:

- Don't let your knees go beyond your toes during the descent.
- Keep your core active to protect your back.
- Distribute your weight evenly on your feet.

Recommended Duration and Repetitions:

- **Repetitions:** Start with 3 sets of 10-15 repetitions each.
- **Rest Between Sets:** Rest for about 30-60 seconds between sets.
- **Frequency:** This exercise can be done 2-3 times a week as part of a leg and core strength training routine.

Single-Leg Squat

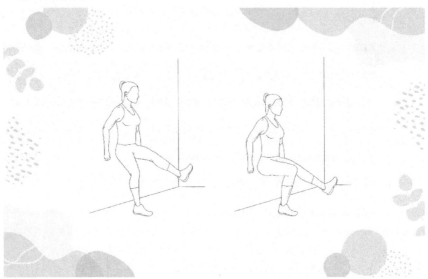

Single-leg squats are particularly effective for improving leg muscle strength and balance, as well as strengthening the glutes. It is a challenging exercise that requires concentration and control and can be a great way to challenge your stability and coordination.

1. **Initial Position:** Stand facing away from the wall. Use the wall for balance by touching it with your hand. One leg will be the supporting leg, while the other remains free and lifted off the ground.
2. **Leg Lift:** Lift the free leg off the ground, keeping it straight in front of you, if possible, or slightly bent at the knee if necessary.
3. **Performing the Squat:** Bend the supporting leg to lower into a one-legged squat as low as possible. Keep your back straight and your chest lifted.

4. **Holding the Position:** Once you are in the lowest position you can maintain, pause briefly.

5. **Returning to Initial Position:** Push through the heel of the supporting leg to return to the initial standing position.

6. **Repetition:** Repeat the exercise for the desired number of repetitions before switching sides.

Tips:

- Focus on balance and control of the movement, especially in the descent and ascent phases.
- Use the wall to help maintain balance but try not to lean too much.
- For beginners, partial squatting can be helpful until more strength and control are developed.

Recommended Duration and Repetitions:

- **Repetitions:** Start with 3 sets of 5-10 repetitions per leg.
- **Rest Between Sets:** Rest for 45-90 seconds between sets.
- **Frequency:** This exercise can be included 1-2 times a week in a leg workout.

Wall Lunges

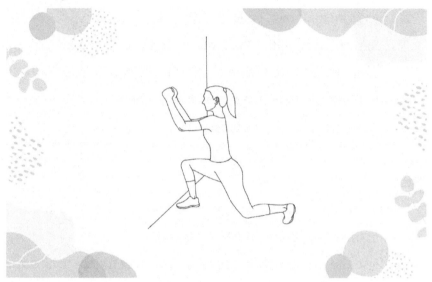

Wall Lunges are an effective exercise for strengthening and toning the glutes and hamstrings, as well as improving balance and coordination. Using the wall for support can help maintain proper posture during the exercise.

1. **Initial Position:** Stand facing the wall, about two feet away. Rest your hands on the wall at shoulder height for support.
2. **Forward Step:** Take a big step forward with your right foot, keeping your left foot in place.
3. **Knee Bend:** Bend both knees to lower your body towards the floor. The front knee (right) should form about a 90-degree angle, and the back knee (left) should almost touch the floor.

4. **Holding the Position:** Keep your torso straight and core active, with your gaze directed towards the wall. Ensure the front knee doesn't go beyond the toe.

5. **Rising Up:** Push on the front heel to return to the upright position. Repeat the movement for the desired number of repetitions.

6. **Switch Legs:** After completing the repetitions with one leg, change and repeat the exercise with your left leg forward.

Tips:

- Keep your hands on the wall for balance if needed.
- Don't let the knee of the advanced leg go beyond the toe.
- Focus on a controlled movement both in the descent and ascent.

Recommended Duration and Repetitions:

- **Repetitions:** Start with 2-3 sets of 8-12 repetitions per leg.
- **Rest Between Sets:** Rest for about 30-60 seconds between sets.
- **Frequency:** You can incorporate this exercise 2-3 times a week as part of a lower limb strength workout.

Wall Bridge

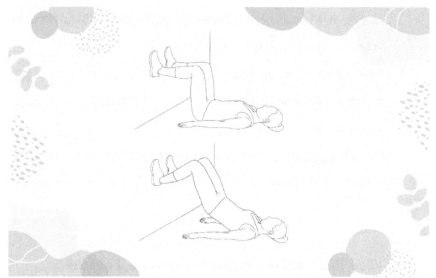

Wall Bridges are particularly beneficial for strengthening glute and core muscles. This wall variant adds a stability and resistance element that can be helpful for those looking to intensify the exercise compared to the traditional floor bridge.

1. **Initial Position:** Lie down on a mat with your legs bent and feet planted against the wall. Your arms are extended along your sides, palms facing down.
2. **Lifting the Hips:** Inhale and lift your hips off the mat by pushing your feet against the wall. Your body should form a straight line from your shoulders to your knees.
3. **Stabilization:** Once in position, squeeze your glutes and hold for a few seconds. Ensure you keep your core stable and avoid overextending your lower back.

4. **Controlled Descent:** Exhale and slowly lower your hips to the mat, vertebra by vertebra, returning to the starting position.
5. **Repeating the Exercise:** Repeat the movement for the desired number of repetitions.

Tips:

- Don't let your hips sag or bend; maintain the straight line of the body during the bridge.
- Focus on pressing your feet against the wall to increase stability and intensity of the exercise.
- Keep the movement fluid and controlled to maximize benefits and reduce the risk of injury.

Recommended Duration and Repetitions:

- **Repetitions:** Start with 2-3 sets of 10-15 repetitions.
- **Rest Between Sets:** Rest for about 30-60 seconds between sets.
- **Frequency:** This exercise can be performed 2-3 times a week as part of a workout for core and glute muscles.

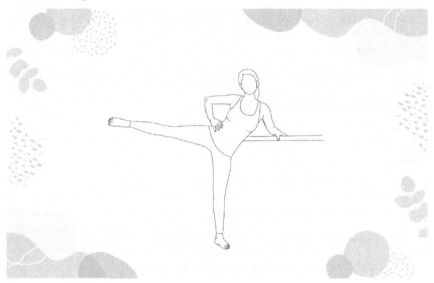

Wall Side Leg Lifts are particularly useful for those aiming to tone and define the sides of the legs and buttocks.

1. **Initial Position:** Stand sideways next to a wall. The hand closest to the wall should rest on it for balance, while the other hand rests on your hip. Your body should be straight, feet together.

2. **Leg Lift:** Slowly lift the leg that's farther from the wall straight out to the side, keeping your foot in a neutral position.

3. **Holding the Position:** Once you reach the maximum height without tilting your torso, hold the position for a second, ensuring the movement is driven by the hip and glute muscles.

4. **Controlled Descent:** Slowly lower the leg, maintaining control, until it returns to the starting position.

5. **Repetition:** Complete the required repetitions on one side before switching and repeating the exercise with the other leg.

Tips:

- Keep your body as straight and stable as possible throughout the exercise.
- Avoid jerky movements or using momentum.
- The working leg should not lift higher than what allows you to maintain stable hips without tilting.

Recommended Duration and Repetitions:

- **Repetitions:** Start with 2-3 sets of 10-12 repetitions per leg.
- **Rest Between Sets:** Rest for about 30 seconds between sets.
- **Frequency:** This exercise can be performed 2-3 times a week, integrating it into a leg or core workout routine.

Wall Calf Raises

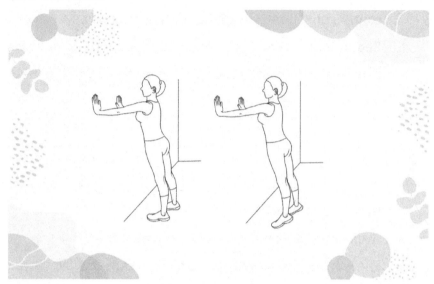

Wall Calf Raises are great for strengthening calf muscles, improving definition, and balance. This exercise is ideal for endurance athletes, people who stand a lot during the day, or anyone who desires more toned and defined legs.

1. **Initial Position:** Stand facing the wall with your feet shoulder-width apart. Your toes should point forward. Lightly rest your hands on the wall for balance.
2. **Lift:** Slowly push onto your tiptoes, raising your heels off the ground as high as possible, as if trying to reach the wall with your head.
3. **Holding the Position:** Once at the top, hold the position for a second, contracting the calf muscles well.

4. **Controlled Descent:** Slowly lower your heels towards the floor without completely touching it, to maintain muscle tension.
5. **Repetition:** Continue performing the lifts for the desired number of repetitions.

Tips:
- Keep your body straight and core active throughout the duration of the exercise.
- Avoid pushing too far forward or backward with your body; the movement should be vertical.
- To increase intensity, perform the exercise on a step or raised surface for greater range of motion.

Recommended Duration and Repetitions:
- **Repetitions:** Perform 3 sets of 15-20 repetitions.
- **Rest Between Sets:** Rest for 30-60 seconds between sets.
- **Frequency:** This exercise can be performed 2-3 times a week as part of a leg workout.

Wall Scissors

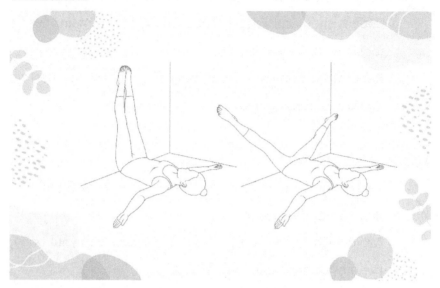

Wall Scissors are optimal for toning the inner and outer thighs and improving hip mobility. This exercise also helps to strengthen abdominal muscles and improve coordination.

1. **Initial Position:** Lie on the floor with your buttocks as close to the wall as possible and legs extended upwards against the wall. Extend your arms outward for greater stability.
2. **Opening:** Slowly open your legs into a wide "V", maintaining contact with the wall. Be careful not to overstretch; you should feel a mild stretch, not pain. Then return to the starting position and repeat.
3. **Control:** Keep the movement controlled and synchronized, without making jerky movements or losing contact with the wall.
4. **Rhythm:** Continue alternating the legs for the duration of the exercise.

5. **Repetition:** Maintain this scissor movement for the recommended number of repetitions.

Tips:

- Keep your core activated to protect your back and increase stability.
- If you feel tension in your lower back, you can slightly bend your knees.
- Maintain steady breathing throughout the exercise, inhaling and exhaling smoothly.

Recommended Duration and Repetitions:

- **Repetitions:** Perform 10 to 15 scissor movements per leg.
- **Sets:** Perform 2 to 3 sets.
- **Rest Between Sets:** Rest for 30 to 60 seconds between sets.
- **Frequency:** This exercise can be performed 2-3 times a week as part of a leg workout or a low-impact cardio routine.

Chapter 6 – Posture Exercises

Wall Posture Check

The "Wall Posture Check" is a great way to restore awareness of correct posture. It's particularly beneficial for those who spend a lot of time sitting or are looking to improve their overall posture. This exercise is more about postural awareness than dynamic movement, so the focus is on understanding your body's alignment in space. You can perform this postural check multiple times throughout the day, especially if you spend many hours seated or in front of a computer.

1. **Initial Position:** Stand with your back against the wall. Your heels should touch the wall, and your arms should be along your sides.

2. **Back Alignment:** Ensure your sacrum (the lower part of your back) and shoulder blades touch the wall. The back of your head should also touch the wall, keeping your chin slightly tucked down to maintain a neutral neck alignment.

3. **Neck Alignment:** Place your hand behind the neck's curve to ensure there is enough space. Your neck should not be flattened against the wall.

4. **Leg Alignment:** Your legs should be straight, and your feet aligned with your shoulders. Your feet should touch the wall

with the heels, while the natural arch of your foot remains slightly lifted off the ground.

5. **Checking Spaces:** There should be a small gap between the wall and your lower back, as well as a small space under the neck's curve.

6. **Holding the Position:** Maintain this position, trying to "lengthen" your spine against the wall without losing contact points. A tip: visualize being "pulled up" by an invisible string from the top of your head to maximize spinal elongation.

7. **Breathing:** While holding the position, take deep breaths and exhale slowly, focusing on maintaining good alignment.

8. **Duration:** Hold the position for 30-60 seconds.

Wall Clock

The "Wall Clock" is an excellent exercise for improving shoulder mobility and strengthening upper body posture awareness. It's ideal for those looking to enhance shoulder flexibility and posture.

1. **Initial Position:** Stand with your back against the wall, feet slightly apart and in line with your shoulders.

2. **Contact with Wall:** Ensure the back of your head, shoulder blades, and sacrum touch the wall. Your arms should be extended along your sides.

3. **Arm Movement:** Raise your arms to the side until they are parallel to the floor, maintaining contact with the wall with your fingers.

4. **Creating the Clock:** Slowly move your arms overhead, as if the hands were clock hands moving upward. Imagine drawing a large circle on the wall with your hands while maintaining contact.

5. **Touching 12 O'Clock:** Once your hands reach the noon position (or as high as possible while maintaining contact with the wall), start bringing your arms back down to the starting position.

6. **Controlled Movement:** The movement should be slow and controlled, being careful to maintain contact with the wall.

7. **Breathing:** Focus on deep, regular breathing throughout the exercise.

Recommended Duration and Repetitions:

- **Duration:** Each "full turn" of the clock should take about 30 seconds.
- **Repetitions:** Perform 3-5 complete clock cycles.
- **Frequency:** You can include this exercise in your daily routine, especially as a break from sedentary work.

Wall Toe Lift

The "Wall Toe Lift" helps to strengthen the muscles of the foot arch and can contribute to improved balance and foot stability.

1. **Initial Position:** Stand with your back straight against the wall, feet flat on the floor, hip-width apart.
2. **Back Against Wall:** Ensure your back, including the lumbar region, maintains light contact with the wall.
3. **Lifting:** Slowly lift your toes while keeping your heels on the ground. Your toes should point upwards as much as possible.
4. **Muscle Tension:** Try to feel the tension along your legs and in the muscles of the foot arch as you lift your toes.
5. **Controlled Release:** Slowly release your toes and bring them back to the floor.
6. **Breathing:** Maintain deep, controlled breathing during the exercise.

Tips:
- **Focus on the sensation of lifting with the muscles of the foot arch, not just the toes.**
- **Keep your heels firm and stable on the ground to better isolate the movement.**

Recommended Duration and Repetitions:
- **Duration:** Hold the toe lift for 2-3 seconds.

- **Repetitions:** Perform 10-15 lifts per set.
- **Sets:** Try doing 2-3 sets.
- **Frequency:** You can do this exercise daily, especially if you're looking to strengthen the foot arch or improve your stability.

Wall March

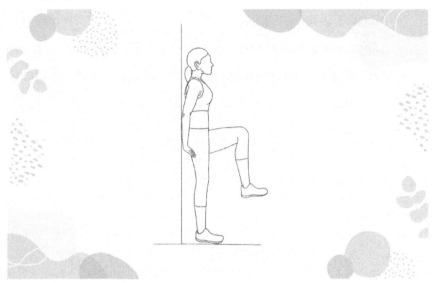

The "Wall March" is an excellent exercise for improving core stability and leg strength, preparing the body for more complex exercises and improving posture and balance.

1. **Initial Position:** Stand with your shoulders against the wall and your hands resting on it, keeping your arms extended and your body straight.

2. **Knee Lift:** Lift one knee at a time, trying to reach a 90-degree angle between the thigh and torso, as if marching in place.

3. **Core Activation:** Keep your abdomen contracted to protect your back and help stabilize the movement.

4. **Breathing:** Inhale as you prepare the movement and exhale during the knee lift.

5. **Controlled Movement:** Ensure you control the movement in both the lifting and lowering phases of the knee. Avoid jerky or overly rapid movements.

Tips:

- Keep your back straight and core active throughout the exercise to prevent lumbar strains.
- Don't push yourself too quickly; the quality of the movement is more important than speed.

Recommended Duration and Repetitions:

- **Duration:** Lift each knee, holding the position for 1-2 seconds before lowering.
- **Repetitions:** Perform 10-15 repetitions per leg.
- **Sets:** Complete 2-3 sets per side.

Chapter 7 – Flexibility Exercises

Hamstring Stretch Against the Wall

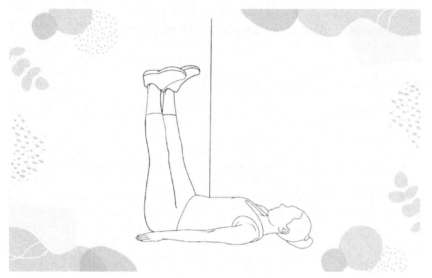

The hamstring stretch at the wall is an excellent exercise to increase flexibility and alleviate tension in the back of the thighs, improving overall mobility and preventing injuries.

1. **Initial Position:** Lie on the floor on your back and position your buttocks as close to a wall as possible.
2. **Leg Extension:** Lift your legs and rest your heels against the wall. Your legs should be straight and perpendicular to your body.
3. **Position Adjustment:** If you feel a strong stretch, adjust your distance from the wall by slightly moving your buttocks backward until the stretch is comfortable yet effective.

4. **Maintaining the Position:** Keep your hands resting on your hips or place them on the floor beside your body for stability.

5. **Breathing:** Maintain deep, regular breathing, trying to relax your hamstring muscles with each exhalation.

6. **Duration of the Stretch:** Hold the position for 20-30 seconds, allowing the weight of your legs and gravity to enhance the stretch.

Tips:

- Ensure your back is straight and in contact with the floor to avoid strains.
- Do not bend your knees; if the stretch is too intense, move slightly away from the wall.
- Do not overstretch to the point of pain.

Recommended Duration and Repetitions:

- **Duration:** Maintain the stretch position for 20-30 seconds.
- **Repetitions:** Repeat the stretch 2-3 times per side, with a short relaxation interval between repetitions.

Chest Stretch

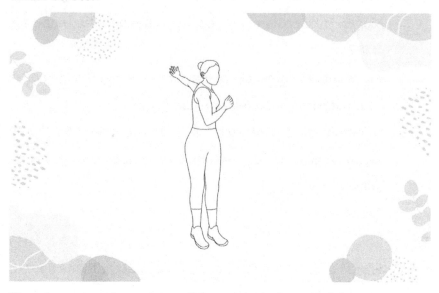

The chest stretch at the wall is particularly useful for countering hunched posture and opening the front of the body, thereby increasing shoulder mobility and reducing tension in the pectoral muscles.

1. **Initial Position:** Stand sideways next to the wall with the arm closest to the wall extended and the hand flat against the surface.
2. **Arm Alignment:** Ensure your arm is at shoulder height and that the palm and forearm are fully in contact with the wall.
3. **Performing the Stretch:** Slowly, rotate your torso away from the wall until you feel a comfortable stretch across the chest and shoulder.

4. **Angle Adjustment:** You can adjust the intensity of the stretch by moving your arm higher or lower along the wall.

5. **Breathing:** Maintain calm, deep breathing, focusing on stretching the pectoral with each exhalation.

6. **Duration of the Stretch:** Hold this position for 20-30 seconds, allowing the chest muscles to relax and stretch.

Tips:

- Do not rotate the body too far from the wall or force the arm; this could cause shoulder tension.
- Use the free hand for balance and support the movement if needed.
- If the stretch is too intense, reduce the angle of body rotation.

Recommended Duration and Repetitions:

- **Duration:** Maintain the stretch position for 20-30 seconds per side.
- **Repetitions:** Repeat the stretch 2-3 times for each side.

Wall Leg Swings

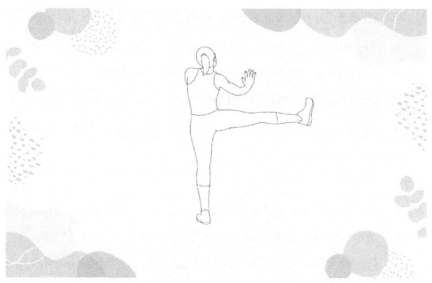

Wall leg swings are excellent for increasing hip movement fluidity, enhancing leg muscle flexibility, and warming up the leg muscles before physical activity.

1. **Initial Position:** Position yourself facing the wall, leaning on it with your hands.
2. **Performing the Swing:** Lift one leg and move it laterally away from your body, then bring it across your center in front of the other leg.
3. **Breathing:** Inhale as you lift the leg and exhale as you bring it back down to the floor or behind you.
4. **Controlled Movement:** Maintain control of the movement during the swing, avoiding using too much momentum.

5. **Maintaining Alignment:** Try to keep your pelvis stable and your torso straight during the swings.

Tips:

- **If you feel excessive tension or pain, reduce the amplitude of the swing.**
- **Keep your knees slightly bent to avoid joint strain.**
- **Focus on hip mobility and core stability.**

Recommended Duration and Repetitions:

- **Duration:** Each swing should last about 2-3 seconds.
- **Repetitions:** Perform 10-15 swings per leg.
- **Sets:** You can do 2-3 sets per side, with a short break between sets.

Wall Spine Stretch

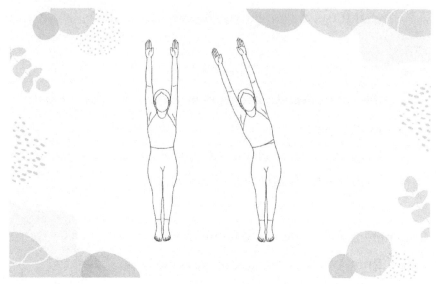

The wall spine stretch helps improve spinal flexibility and relax back muscles, which is beneficial for those who spend many hours seated or experience tension in the lower back.

1. **Initial Position:** Stand with your back facing the wall, feet shoulder-width apart and slightly away from the wall. Raise your arms upward.
2. **Wall Contact:** Ensure the upper part of your back and your buttocks touch the wall.
3. **Movement:** Slide your arms down the wall and bend your torso to the right.
4. **Maintaining the Position:** Reach the maximum point of inclination and hold this position.
5. **Breathing:** Focus on slow and deep breathing, trying to further relax your back with each exhalation.

6. **Returning to Initial Position:** Slowly return to the starting position while maintaining contact with the wall. Repeat the movement, sliding to the left this time.

Recommended Duration and Repetitions:

- **Duration:** Hold the stretch for 15-30 seconds.
- **Repetitions:** You can repeat the stretch 2-3 times.
- **Sets:** Typically, one set is sufficient, but you can add more sets if you feel particularly stiff.

Shoulder Stretch Against the Wall

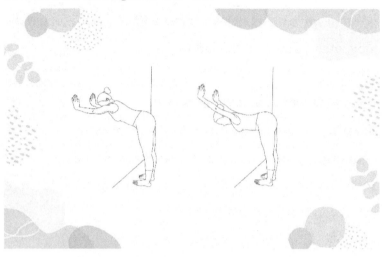

1. **Initial Position:** Stand facing the wall, torso slightly bent, arms extended, and hands against the wall as if pushing it.

2. **Movement:** As you slide your hands upward, lower your torso further and slightly bow your head down.

3. **Maintaining the Position:** Once you reach a comfortable stretch, hold the position. Ensure the rest of your body is relaxed and the shoulder doesn't lift towards the ear.

4. **Breathing:** Take deep breaths and with each exhalation, try to further relax the shoulder, increasing the stretch if possible.

5. **Returning to Initial Position:** Return to the starting position by sliding your hands down and lifting your torso.

Recommended Duration and Repetitions:

- **Duration:** Hold the stretch for 20-30 seconds per side.
- **Repetitions:** You can repeat the stretching 2-3 times.

74

Knee to Chest Stretch

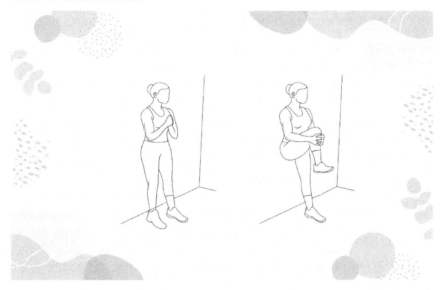

This type of stretching helps improve flexibility in the lower back and hips. It's also beneficial for relaxing muscles after prolonged sitting or intense workouts.

1. **Initial Position:** Stand with your back to the wall. Ensure your buttocks, head, and upper back are well-pressed against the wall.

2. **Bringing Knee to Chest:** Choose one leg to work on first. Using your hands, grasp the knee of that leg and gently pull it toward your chest, keeping the other leg straight and pressed against the wall.

3. **Stretch:** Continue pulling the knee toward your chest until you feel a comfortable stretch in the lower back and along the hip muscles of the bent leg.

4. **Breathing:** Maintain slow, deep breathing, trying to relax further with each exhalation.

5. **Duration of the Stretch:** Hold this position for 20-30 seconds per leg, feeling the stretch and release of tension.

6. **Repetition:** Slowly release the leg, extend it along the wall, and repeat the stretch with the other leg.

Recommended Duration and Repetitions:

- **Duration:** Maintain the stretch for 20-30 seconds per leg.
- **Repetitions:** Perform the stretch 2-3 times for each leg.
- **Frequency:** Can be practiced daily to promote flexibility and relaxation of lumbar and hip muscles.

Chapter 8 – 28-day challenge

How it works

The 28-Day Challenge is designed as a comprehensive workout program that incorporates a variety of exercises discussed earlier. The goal is to reshape your body, tone your muscles, and enhance overall well-being, making you feel rejuvenated by the end of the 28-day period. The exercises have been thoughtfully mixed and structured to gradually increase in difficulty, ensuring a balanced approach to fitness.

Here's how the challenge works:

Structure

1. **Daily Workouts:** Each day, you will have a specific set of exercises to perform. These exercises will be a mix of flexibility, posture, and strength training, taken from the exercises we discussed.

2. **Progressive Difficulty:** The workouts will progressively become more challenging each week. This gradual increase helps your body adapt and grow stronger without overwhelming it.

3. **Repetitions and Duration:** Each exercise's repetition and duration have been carefully selected to optimize results. It's important to follow these guidelines closely.

Guidelines

1. **Consistency:** Perform the workouts daily. Consistency is key to seeing results.

2. **Hydration and Nutrition:** Drink plenty of water and maintain a balanced diet to fuel your body for the workouts.

3. **Warm-up:** Before starting the workout, dedicate 5 minutes to a general warm-up which can include marching in place, arm circles, and mobilization of the neck and spine.

4. **Breathing:** Ensure you maintain controlled breathing and execute each movement with precision rather than speed.

5. **Rest:** For this specific program, consistently maintain a rest period of 30 seconds between each set of the same exercise and 50 seconds of rest between different exercises.

6. **Workout duration.** Each day, simply follow the exercises outlined in the workout sheets provided in the subsequent pages. Super simple and super quick! But, depending on your time availability and physical condition, you may consider repeating the same workout up to 5 times per day. This means that after completing the last exercise listed in the worksheet for that specific day, you'll take a 50-second rest and then you'll start again from the first exercise. Naturally, this process can significantly enhance your results.

7. **When:** The ideal times to perform your wall Pilates session are in the late afternoon before dinner, or early in the morning. Depending on your schedule and physical capacity, you might consider doubling your workout sessions – one in the early morning and another in the late

evening. Each session should consist of one complete workout, as described in the tables below, and you can do up to 5 repetitions of this workout per session, as mentioned earlier.

Monitoring Progress

- **Journaling:** Keep a workout journal to track your progress, noting how you felt each day and the repetitions you completed.
- **Photographs:** Taking weekly photographs can be a motivating way to visually track your progress.
- **Reflect on Well-being:** Regularly assess how you feel overall – improvements in energy levels, mood, and physical fitness are key indicators of your progress.

Post-Challenge

After completing the 28 days, evaluate your progress. Remember that the journey to fitness is ongoing, and this challenge is just a step toward a longer, healthier lifestyle. You could consider repeating the challenge, perhaps varying the exercises and/or increasing the intensity (in terms of number/duration of repetitions).

Daily Workouts

Monday: Upper Body and Core

Exercise	Repetitions/Duration	Sets
Wall Push-up	12-15	2
Wall Angel	12-15	2
Wall Crunch	12-15	2
Wall Plank	30 sec	2
Wall Rowing	12-15	2
Wall Sit	30 sec	2

Tuesday: Legs and Flexibility

Exercise	Repetitions/Duration	Sets
Wall Squat	15	2
Lateral Leg Lift	12 per leg	2
Wall Calf Raises	15	2
Hamstring Stretch	30 sec per leg	2
Wall Leg Swing	10 per leg	2
Wall Posture Check	30 sec	2

Wednesday: Core and Stability

Exercise	Repetitions/Duration	Sets
Wall Hundred	100 (short pulses)	1
Reverse Wall Plank	30 sec	2
Wall Sit with Knee Raise	30 sec	2
Wall Teaser	8	2
Side Wall Crunch	12 per side	2
Wall Bridge	12	2

Thursday: Endurance and Posture

Exercise	Repetitions/Duration	Sets
Single Arm Wall Push-up	8 per arm	2
Knee Fold Wall Plank	12 per side	2
Wall Clock	30 sec	2
One-Legged Wall Squat	8 per leg	2
Wall Shoulder Stretch	30 sec per side	2
Wall Marching	30 sec	2

Friday: Strength and Mobility

Exercise	Repetitions/Duration	Sets
Wall Roll-Ups	10	2
Wall Lunges	10 per leg	2
Rear Leg Lift	12 per leg	2
Wall Scissors	12 per side	2
Wall Chest Stretch	30 sec per side	2
Wall Toe Lift	15	2

Saturday: Full Body

Exercise	Repetitions/Duration	Sets
Wall Push-up	12-15	2
Wall Bridge	12	2
Wall Teaser	8	2
Wall Lunges	10 per leg	2
Wall Leg Swing	10 per leg	2
Wall Spine Stretch	30 sec	2

Sunday: Rest or Low-Intensity Activity Use Sunday for rest or to engage in low-intensity activities such as walking, light yoga, or swimming.

For the next week, we can change the order and intensity of the exercises to continue stimulating the body and prevent monotony.

Monday: Core and Posture

Exercise	Repetitions/Duration	Sets
Wall Plank	40 sec	3
Wall Hundred	100 (short bursts)	1
Wall Sit with Knee Raise	40 sec	3
Wall Clock	40 sec	3
Wall Teaser	10	3
Wall Posture Check	40 sec	3

Tuesday: Endurance and Flexibility

Exercise	Repetitions/Duration	Sets
Wall Push-up	15-20	3
Wall Scissors	15 per side	3
One-Legged Squat	10 per leg	3
Wall Spine Stretch	40 sec	3
Wall Chest Stretch	40 sec per side	3
Wall Leg Swing	12 per leg	3

Wednesday: Strength and Stability

Exercise	Repetitions/Duration	Sets
Single Arm Wall Push-up	10 per arm	3
Reverse Wall Plank	40 sec	3
Wall Bridge	15	3
Wall Roll-Ups	12	3
Wall Toe Lift	20	3
Side Wall Crunch	15 per side	3

Thursday: Leg and Core Strengthening

Exercise	Repetitions/Duration	Sets
Wall Squat	20	3
Wall Lunges	12 per leg	3
Wall Calf Raises	20	3
Wall Sit	45 sec	3
Knee Fold Wall Plank	15 per side	3
Wall Crunch	15	3

Friday: Balance and Body Control

Exercise	Repetitions/Duration	Sets
Wall Angel	15-20	3
Lateral Leg Lift	15 per leg	3
Rear Leg Lift	15 per leg	3
Wall Marching	45 sec	3
Wall Shoulder Stretch	40 sec per side	3
Knee to Chest	12 per leg	3

Saturday: Full Body Mix

Exercise	Repetitions/Duration	Sets
Wall Rowing	20	3
Wall Scissors	16 per side	3
Wall Bridge	15	3
Wall Roll-Ups	12	3
Hamstring Stretch	40 sec per side	3
Side Wall Crunch	15 per side	3

Sunday: Rest or Low-Intensity Activity The rest day is crucial for muscle recovery. You can dedicate it to total relaxation or a low-intensity activity such as yoga, walking, or light swimming.

Week 3

This program continues to vary the exercises and intensity to prevent excessive adaptation and to keep the body in a state of continuous improvement.

Monday: Core Strength and Stability

Exercise	Repetitions/Duration	Sets
Wall Teaser	10	3
Wall Sit with Knee Raise	45 sec	3
Reverse Wall Plank	45 sec	3
Wall Hundred	100 (short bursts)	1
Wall Roll-Ups	15	3
Side Wall Crunch	20 per side	3

Tuesday: Upper Body Strengthening

Exercise	Repetitions/Duration	Sets
Wall Push-up	20	3
Wall Rowing	20	3
Wall Angel	20	3
Single Arm Wall Push-up	12 per arm	3
Wall Shoulder Stretch	45 sec per side	3
Wall Posture Check	45 sec	3

Wednesday: Leg Focus

Exercise	Repetitions/Duration	Sets
Wall Squat	25	3
One-Legged Squat	12 per leg	3
Wall Calf Raises	25	3
Wall Lunges	15 per leg	3
Wall Scissors	20 per side	3
Wall Bridge	18	3

Thursday: Advanced Core and Posture

Exercise	Repetitions/Duration	Sets
Knee Fold Wall Plank	18 per side	3
Wall Clock	45 sec	3
Wall Sit	50 sec	3
Wall Crunch	20	3
Wall Toe Lift	25	3
Wall Marching	50 sec	3

Friday: Endurance and Flexibility

Exercise	Repetitions/Duration	Sets
Wall Leg Swing	15 per leg	3
Hamstring Stretch	45 sec per side	3
Chest Stretch	45 sec per side	3
Wall Spine Stretch	45 sec	3
Wall Squat	25	3
Wall Posture Check	50 sec	3

Saturday: Dynamic Full Body Mix

Exercise	Repetitions/Duration	Sets
Wall Push-up	20	3
Lateral Leg Lift	20 per leg	3
Wall Bridge	20	3
Wall Hundred	100 (short bursts)	1
Wall Plank	50 sec	3
Wall Lunges	15 per leg	3

Sunday: Active Recovery or Rest

Yoga, deep stretching, or a relaxing walk to promote muscle recovery.

Week 4

This workout plan intensifies the sessions by increasing the number of repetitions and sets and strategically combining exercises to maximize strength and stability training.

Monday: Upper Body and Core Strengthening

Exercise	Repetitions/Duration	Sets
Wall Push-up	20	4
Single Arm Wall Push-up	10 per arm	4
Wall Angel	20	4
Wall Rowing	20	4
Side Wall Crunch	20 per side	4
Wall Roll-Ups	15	4

Tuesday: Legs and Stability

Exercise	Repetitions/Duration	Sets
Wall Squat	25	4
One-Legged Squat	15 per leg	3
Wall Lunges	20 per leg	4
Wall Bridge	20	4
Rear Leg Lift	20 per leg	3
Wall Calf Raises	25	4

Wednesday: Intensive Core

Exercise	Repetitions/Duration	Sets
Wall Plank	60 sec	4
Knee Fold Wall Plank	15 per side	4
Reverse Wall Plank	60 sec	4
Wall Teaser	15	4
Wall Crunch	20	4
Wall Hundred	100 (short bursts)	2

Thursday: Upper Body and Posture

Exercise	Repetitions/Duration	Sets
Wall Push-up	25	4
Single Arm Wall Push-up	12 per arm	3
Wall Angel	25	4
Wall Rowing	25	4
Wall Posture Check	60 sec	3
Wall Clock	60 sec	3

Friday: Legs and Flexibility

Exercise	Repetitions/Duration	Sets
Wall Squat	30	4
Wall Lunges	25 per leg	4
Wall Bridge	25	4
Wall Calf Raises	30	4
Hamstring Stretch	60 sec per side	3
Wall Leg Swing	20 per leg	3

Saturday: Dynamic Full Body

Exercise	Repetitions/Duration	Sets
Wall Push-up	30	3
Side Wall Crunch	25 per side	3
One-Legged Squat	18 per leg	3
Lateral Leg Lift	20 per leg	3
Reverse Wall Plank	70 sec	3
Wall Scissors	25 per side	3

Sunday: Active Recovery or Rest

Recovery activities like light stretching, yoga, walking, or other types of low-intensity mobility to promote muscle relaxation.

Bonus Chapter- Breathing and Relaxation Techniques

Welcome to a special bonus section of our book, dedicated to the art of breathing and relaxation. We've included this as a gift to you, our readers, recognizing the immense value these practices can add to your overall well-being.

Breathing and relaxation are more than just mere exercises; they are transformative experiences that can be woven into the fabric of your daily life. When paired with your Pilates workouts, these techniques not only enhance the effectiveness of each session but also elevate your sense of well-being to new heights.

We'll explore various breathing and relaxation methods that are easy to integrate into any moment of your day. Whether you're amidst a busy schedule, taking a break at work, or winding down before bed, these practices are your tools for maintaining balance and harmony. They can transform not just your Pilates practice, but your entire approach to life, contributing significantly to a higher state of health and happiness.

Breathing Techniques

Practicing these breathing techniques before starting your Pilates session can help focus, relax the body, and mentally and physically prepare for the exercises. Always remember to listen to your body and adjust the pace of your breathing so that it best supports your movement during Pilates practice. Breathing in Pilates is crucial because it supports movement, helps control the execution of exercises, and increases the effectiveness of the work on the core.

Diaphragmatic or Abdominal Breathing
1. **Position:** Lie on your back with your knees bent and feet flat on the ground. You can put one hand on your abdomen and the other on your chest to feel the movement of your breath.
2. **Breathing:** While inhaling, focus on expanding the diaphragm downwards. You'll feel your abdomen rise under your hand, while the hand on your chest remains relatively still.
3. **Exhalation:** Exhale slowly through your mouth, as if you were blowing through a straw, feeling your abdomen lower and the core activate.
4. **Rhythm:** Maintain a regular and controlled rhythm. The duration of the exhalation should be slightly longer than the inhalation.

Lateral or Thoracic Breathing
1. **Position:** Sit up straight or remain in the supine position.
2. **Breathing:** While inhaling, focus on expanding the sides of your ribcage, rather than the chest or abdomen.
3. **Exhalation:** Exhale through your mouth, feeling your ribcage draw back towards the spine.

4. **Rhythm:** Ensure you maintain a fluid breath and do not hold your breath. Complete Breathing

5. **Position:** Standing, sitting, or lying down, with the spine in a neutral position.

6. **Breathing:** Combining both abdominal and thoracic breathing, start inhaling and lifting the abdomen first and then expanding the ribcage.

7. **Exhalation:** Begin to exhale from the chest and then the abdomen, emptying the lungs completely and activating the core.

8. **Rhythm:** The breath should be calm and controlled, without haste or shortness.

Rhythmic Breathing for Movement

1. **Position:** Any position that will be used in the following exercises.

2. **Breathing:** Coordinate your breath with the movement, generally inhaling during the preparation phase of the movement and exhaling during the execution of the more intense exercise or when greater strength is required.

3. **Exhalation:** Use the exhalation to assist in the movement and in activating the core, especially during movements that require stability and control.

4. **Rhythm:** The rhythm of your breath should follow that of the movement, creating a constant and rhythmic flow that supports the exercise.

Relaxation Techniques

Incorporating these techniques into your Pilates routine or daily life can significantly impact your physical and mental well-being. Loosening muscles and calming the mind before exercising helps prepare the body to move more effectively, while post-workout relaxation is vital for optimal recovery. But the benefits of these techniques don't stop there; they can also be a lifesaver during tense moments throughout the day, helping manage stress and improve sleep quality. Through relaxation, we can achieve an emotional balance that is an integral part of a holistic approach to well-being. This state of balance is essential for maintaining focus and attention during Pilates exercises, performing them with greater precision and care. Moreover, when the body is relaxed, the breathing process becomes more efficient, making the most of diaphragm capacity and improving overall oxygenation.

The benefits are endless:
- **Reduce Stress:** Relaxation helps calm the mind, reducing cortisol levels, the stress hormone.
- **Improve Circulation:** Relaxation techniques can enhance blood circulation, facilitating the transport of oxygen and nutrients to the muscles.
- **Prevent Injuries:** A relaxed body is less susceptible to injuries, as tense or contracted muscles are more prone to tears and strains.
- **Increase Body Awareness:** Being relaxed allows for greater awareness of one's physical condition, enhancing the ability to perceive and correct posture.

Jacobson's Progressive Relaxation

Jacobson's Progressive Relaxation is a technique developed by American physician Edmund Jacobson in the 1920s. Benefits of this practice include stress and anxiety reduction, improved sleep, decreased blood pressure, muscle relaxation, and improved concentration. Jacobson believed that if people could learn to voluntarily relax their muscles, they could significantly reduce their anxiety levels. Through his technique, one learns to distinguish between feelings of tension and complete relaxation and, over time, reduce chronic muscle tension.

How to Practice:

1. **Find a Quiet Environment:** Start by finding a quiet place where you won't be disturbed. Lie on the floor or sit comfortably in a chair with back support. Close your eyes to eliminate visual distractions.

2. **Focus on Muscle Groups:** The technique proceeds by individually working on each muscle group of the body. Initially, you might focus on the muscles of the hands, then move on to arms, shoulders, neck, and so on, down to the feet.

3. **Tension and Relaxation:** Focus on one muscle group at a time. Tense the muscles in question (e.g., clenching your fist or flexing your foot) and maintain this tension for about five seconds, being careful not to reach the point of causing pain or cramps.

4. **Conscious Relaxation:** After maintaining tension, release the muscle group with a slow exhalation, paying attention to the sensation of relaxation that follows. You should try to

feel the difference between the states of tension and relaxation.

5. **Wait and Transition:** After releasing the tension, wait about 15-20 seconds before moving to the next muscle group. This pause allows you to savor the feeling of relaxation and prepares the body and mind for the next step.

6. **Progression:** Continue the process for all muscle groups of the body, generally starting from the head and moving towards the feet or vice versa. This progressive method helps to systematically relax the entire body.

7. **Breathing:** Breathing plays a key role in progressive relaxation. During the exercises, you should use deep, controlled breathing to increase the relaxing effect.

8. **Regularity:** Regular practice of Jacobson's Progressive Relaxation can enhance its benefits. Over time, it becomes easier to recognize tension areas in the body and relax them more quickly.

9. **Body Awareness:** As you become more skilled in the technique, you'll develop a greater awareness of your bodily sensations and be able to relax muscles even without the preliminary tension.

Meditation or Mindfulness

Mindfulness, or attentive awareness, is a form of meditation that emphasizes awareness of the present moment. Instead of focusing on a specific object or thought, mindfulness encourages the practitioner to observe all aspects of the current experience without judgment, whether thoughts, sounds, bodily sensations, or emotions. How to Practice Mindfulness:

1. **Attentive Observation:** Pay attention to the details of your immediate experience, like the sensation of air on your skin, background noise, your thoughts, or emotions that emerge and fade away.
2. **Acceptance:** Embrace each experience without trying to change it. This includes negative thoughts or uncomfortable emotions, observing them with detachment and without automatically reacting.
3. **Return to the Present:** When your mind starts to wander into the past or future, gently bring your attention back to the present moment.
4. **Daily Practice:** Mindfulness can be practiced at any time, not just during a formal meditation session but also while performing daily activities.

Passive Stretching

Passive stretching is a technique where the muscle is extended to the point of maximum tension and held in that position for a certain period without the subject's active involvement. Unlike active stretching, where the subject uses their strength to perform the stretch, in passive stretching an external agent (which can be another person, gravity, or an accessory like a band or towel) helps apply the necessary pressure to increase the stretch. Here's how to practice passive stretching:

1. **Choose the Muscle to Stretch:** Decide which muscle or muscle group you want to stretch. This could be based on a

specific need, like stiffness in a particular body area, or part of a general stretching routine.

2. **Starting Position:** Assume a starting position that allows the target muscle to relax. For example, to stretch the hamstring muscles, you might sit with your legs extended in front of you.

3. **Apply Tension:** Once in position, use an external agent to apply a force that stretches the muscle. This can be done with the help of a partner who gently pushes the body into a greater stretching position, or you can use your body weight or an accessory.

4. **Maintain the Stretch:** The stretch is held passively, without contracting the muscle, for a period ranging from 15 seconds to several minutes. It's important to breathe deeply and maintain relaxation during this time.

5. **Repeat if Necessary:** After maintaining the stretch for the desired time, slowly release the tension and, if necessary, repeat the stretch for more sets.

Guided Visualization

With your eyes closed, imagine a peaceful and serene place. Visualize yourself performing fluid and relaxed movements, exploring the sensation of lightness and peace.

Autogenic Training

Autogenic training is a form of relaxation therapy developed by German psychiatrist Johannes Heinrich Schultz in the 1920s. Schultz discovered that his patients who practiced hypnosis could enter a state of deep relaxation with specific physical sensations. Inspired by this discovery, he developed a method that people could use to self-induce these relaxation conditions without a hypnotist's help. Autogenic training is based on autogenic concentration, i.e., the individual focuses on physical sensations, leading the body into a state of relaxation and ease. The method is systematic and standardized, consisting of exercises that progressively induce a sense of calm and relaxation throughout the body. The practice of autogenic training begins with exercises that focus attention on certain bodily sensations, such as the weight of the limbs or warmth in different body parts.

There are various sequences of exercises that focus on:

Weight: Feeling heavy increases the sensation of muscle relaxation.

Warmth: Perceiving warmth throughout the body promotes vasodilation and relaxation.

Heartbeat: Focusing on the heartbeat can lead to greater internal harmony and calm.

Breathing: Being aware of natural breathing helps relax the nervous system.

Abdominal Warmth: Concentrating on warmth in the abdominal region promotes internal relaxation.

Cool Forehead: Imagining coolness on the forehead can help keep the mind clear and calm. In the exercise, repetitive self-suggestion formulas are used, like "my arms are very heavy," which the individual mentally repeats to facilitate the relaxation process. Sitting or lying down, focus on different body parts and mentally "tell" those parts to relax. You might start with your feet, saying "my feet are heavy and calm," and proceed along the entire body.

Extra Content

Join us on an exclusive journey!

Uncover a treasure trove of extra content and additional resources

waiting for you to explore and enjoy.

- Guided meditations
- Relaxing Music
- Nature sounds for anxiety relief
- ...and much more!

Scan the QR-code or follow the link below to access everything:

https://www.readingroadspress.com/wall-pilates-bonus

Printed in Great Britain
by Amazon

38885894R00056